80% of foam mats are unknowingly ill parents

---How to buy non-toxic alphabet puzzle mat

Author: Hebai

Friday, August 16, 2019

Recommended resources

----

https://amzn.to/2ZXoBIC

SAFEST Non Toxic Alphabet Puzzle Mat

Http://tomhua.com/cn/v/aff/aff.php?affid=17571

E-commerce treasure box

Http://wischina.cn/dvd/?affid=17571

World Internet Summit full video DVD

Http://wischina.cn/faba/lp2/?affid=17571

Send Bar Enterprise Edition

Http://www.ctrip.com/?AllianceID=108078
5&sid=2061295&ouid=&app=0101F00

Ctrip

The cosmetics store sales speech (electronic version), which was first revealed, immediately improved the overall quality of store employees, and the sales of 500+ stores surged by more than 50%...

https://k.weidian.com/zVbKtM6A

Beauty salon front store backyard extension method collection (electronic version), so that the store no longer lacks customers, immediately upgrade store customers 50+ monthly

https://k.weidian.com/bLbPpL4j

If you don't know this technology in the future, what I want to say is that your business will be very difficult. It can be said that this technology is the fastest money-making skill in the world. If you don't understand it, you can only blame God for unfairness every day. Why is the situation as I said? Click to get: Https://share.lizhiweike.com/channel/522649?st=sharelink&inviter_id=66402134&share_platform=app

Chuanglan 253 Cloud Service

Http://cps.253.com/redirect/url?did=386&rid=0&jump=http://zz.253.com/site/register.html

Susie shop

https://m.sudian178.com/#/weex/gift-

list?investCode=266331545&isShare=1&fro
m=singlemessage

**PS Tutorial Super Compilation [1000
episodes of Champion]**

https://study.163.com/course/introduction
/1442008.htm?share=1&shareId=13975402
43

**AI Tutorial Super Compilation [500+
Champion Class]**

(https://study.163.com/course/introductio
n/1003241018.htm?share=1&shareId=1397
540243

**AE Tutorial Super Compilation [400+
Champion Class]**

(https://study.163.com/course/introductio

n/1005103011.htm?share=1&shareId=1397
540243

With Jian Qi Xuecai

(https://study.163.com/course/introductio
n/1003418002.htm?share=1&shareId=1397
540243

**Easy to learn hand-drawn for the workplace
plus points**

(https://study.163.com/course/introductio
n/1003373019.htm?share=1&shareId=1397
540243

**26 PPT practical classes thoroughly open the
production thinking**

(https://study.163.com/course/introductio

n/1006225007.htm?share=1&shareId=1397
540243

Product Manager - Methodology + Actual Combat

(https://study.163.com/course/introductio
n/1003240007.htm?share=1&shareId=1397
540243

Soft Text Master - Marketing Copywriting Cheats

(https://study.163.com/course/introductio
n/1665014.htm?share=1&shareId=1397540
243

How does the income from wages go from 0 to 100,000 per month

(https://study.163.com/course/introductio
n/1005577007.htm?share=1&shareId=1397
540243

Efficient learning: Cheats for double the value of the workplace

(https://study.163.com/course/introductio
n/1004627006.htm?share=1&shareId=1397
540243

How to effectively improve your workplace influence

(https://study.163.com/course/introductio
n/1005530009.htm?share=1&shareId=1397
540243

MBA management class entrance exam (logical series) weakened strengthen

(https://m.ke.qq.com/course/434685?saleToken=1726006&saleLink&from=h5link

MBA PubMed English II (translation and writing)

(https://m.ke.qq.com/course/432482?saleToken=1726007&saleLink&from=h5link

2019 Institutional Public Basic Knowledge Innovation Course

(https://m.ke.qq.com/course/433170?saleToken=1726008&saleLink&from=h5link

188 sentences of universal travel

(https://m.ke.qq.com/course/434061?saleToken=1726013&saleLink&from=h5link

"Standard Japanese 1" full course

(https://m.ke.qq.com/course/402122?saleToken=1726016&saleLink&from=h5link

Seoul Korean Extraordinary Series Elementary (TOPIK1~TOPIK2)

(https://m.ke.qq.com/course/402349?saleToken=1726018&saleLink&from=h5link

German original textbook "Begegnungen" famous teacher (A2)

(https://m.ke.qq.com/course/413014?saleToken=1726023&saleLink&from=h5link

AEIS/IELTS/TOEFL English exam preparation will be grammatical (https://m.ke.qq.com/course/421352?saleToken=1726026&saleLink&from=h5link

The National Second Construction Examination Management is full of the 2004 issue (https://m.ke.qq.com/course/433298?saleToken=1726030&saleLink&from=h5link

Zero-based piano speed learning 10 songs for 100 minutes (https://study.163.com/course/introduction/1006551009.htm?share=1&shareId=1397540243

Zero-based yoga stretching, giving a fake neck

(https://study.163.com/course/introduction/1004850001.htm?share=1&shareId=1397540243

7 minutes fat burning exercise - 28 days full version

(https://study.163.com/course/introduction/1005229016.htm?share=1&shareId=1397540243

Freelance photographer

http://163.lu/QZ4G73

Real Estate Data Analyst

http://163.lu/xNYfY1

Machine Learning Engineer

http://163.lu/oqoGu0

New Media Video Director

http://163.lu/PfMMl4

Applicable regulations

The book was published in 2019, copyright is owned by Hebai, and ownership is protected. No part of this publication may be reproduced or stored in a retrieval system without the written consent of the copyright holder, and may not be reproduced in any form by electronic, magazine, photocopying, recording or any other form. No one can give any part of the book to others in any way. Only current members who purchase this book may sell this book and, in accordance with the Terms of Use, no one may donate or sell the book to others through eBay or any form of auction.

Disclaimer

The opinions of this book do not apply to everyone. The message in this book is based on the author's own belief in reliable channels and his personal experience, but the author does not give the reader any hints to ensure the accuracy of the content of this book. Authors, publishers and distributors have never given readers any professional advice on the legal, financial, medical and other fields. Readers are advised by more authoritative experts who will provide you with reasonable advice based on what you have learned. The author, publisher, and supplier of this book do not assume the debt, loss, or risk caused by the reader's personal direct or indirect actions on the content of this book. Any reader must bear full responsibility for what he or she has done after reading this book. All the images that appear in this book are for reference only. The characters in the book have nothing to do with the book, the author and the publisher. This book does not imply any connection between characters, nor is the reader free to guess. All images are licensed for this book and may not be used without the consent of the copyright holder.

about the author

Hebai, the author of this book. More than ten years of offline operation experience, this article is the author's many years of experience, I hope to help you. For more details, please pay attention to the WeChat public account: Hebai Marketing Research Institute (bhyx365).

table of Contents

Recently, many media have reported that foam plastic mats have been banned in Belgium and France, because the mat will release a toxic substance, formamide, which will harm children's health.

The reporter visited a physical store that sells baby products and found that such puzzle mats have been hotly sold in China. What is worrying is that many parents are still not aware of the dangers of this foam puzzle mat.

Alphabet puzzle pad helps children learn the advantages

Of course, books are also fun, but they are nothing compared to a fascinating, cute and exciting alphabet puzzle pad! Now your little one can learn new words and learn how to calculate and have fun!

Puzzle mat or harmful skin

Recently, a survey conducted by the Belgian "Shopping Testing" Association showed that plastic mats commonly used by children use a substance called formamide to make it soft during production. If it is inhaled or swallowed, it will

cause harm to the eyes and The skin is also damaged. Therefore, the country suspended the sale of foam puzzle mats. Subsequently, France also announced a moratorium on the sale of foam puzzle mats for three months.
In China, many merchants are selling foam puzzle mats for children. According to the salesman of a baby store in Yanjiang Road, the foam puzzle mat can be used for a variety of things, floor mats, jigsaw puzzles, soft blocks, and some good quality can also be used as a yoga mat, so the sales are very good.

When the reporter asked if the quality of these mats was guaranteed, the sales staff raised their tips and said that the products were all obtained from the formal channels without worrying about quality problems, but she refused to unpack and let the reporters see the goods. Later, the reporter came to the trade city and found that almost all the shops selling student stationery were sold with such puzzle mats. Apart from the wide variety of prices, the manufacturers of these mats are

different, and the thickness and hardness are not the same. .
Since some of the floor mats sold here did not have a child-specific logo, the reporter asked the owner of a stationery store. The boss replied: "You like how to use it, and you can use it for anyone." The reporter picked up a piece of jigsaw puzzle that had been packaged and smelled a lot of plastic. Asked the boss, I was told that I just started using it. "It doesn't exist when you use it."

Do not know the floor mat hazard

" Climbing on the mat is fast, and the colorful picture can stimulate the brain development of the child." Ms. Cao, who just bought the mat for her baby, told the reporter that the mothers around her almost bought the mat for the baby. Some are puzzle-style, and some are a whole piece. "The seller told me that this is imported, non-toxic and tasteless." Many mothers said that the first factor to consider when purchasing the mat is whether the material is environmentally friendly, but what kind of mat is used. Environmental protection is not very clear, only listen to the seller. Another 80-year-old mother, Miss Li, told reporters that she had bought two sets of jigsaw mats at home. Because she was afraid of too many bacteria, her family often washed them, but they all faded, and I smelled a thorn before the washing. The taste of the nose, after a few washes, the taste slowly fades. After that, Miss Li no longer bought this kind of puzzle for the children. "Because children have long teeth and like to pick things up, if they pick up the mat, they feel very dangerous."

The reporter saw in the online store that the children's plastic mats currently on the market are available in EVA and PE. The price ranges from a few dollars to several hundred yuan. The general puzzle mats are mostly EVA materials. Most of the floor mats are made of PE material, and almost all products are called "non-toxic and tasteless". The reporter asked a seller online whether the product in his store contained formamide. The store said that he did not know what formamide was. More sellers are avoiding reporters' questions.

Large supermarkets, quality platform purchases are more secure

It is reported that most countries have not yet developed standards for the identification of such products as children's plastic puzzle mats, so the impact on the domestic market cannot be assessed. Dong Jinshi, secretary general of the International Food Packaging Association and plastics expert, told the media that the cost of foam plastic mats produced in countries around the world is basically similar.

Therefore, the practice of selling in Belgium and France should also attract the attention of parents in various countries and try to make children use less.

According to reports, the use of formamide in foamed plastic products has two functions. One is to foam the plastic. The larger the amount, the lighter the plastic, the lower the production cost. The second is to increase the flexibility of the plastic product, making it not easy. fracture. However, this kind of thing is a carcinogen, and it is necessary to control the amount of use. Because the current regulations on foamed plastic products at home and abroad do not restrict the amount of formamide used, some manufacturers have increased their use from their own interests. If this phenomenon is a wind, it will be a great hazard to consumers, so it should attract the attention of relevant departments.

Does the foam EVA floor mat smell great, is it toxic?

Foam EVA mats are generally foamed from EVA plastic. The EVA raw material needs to be added with a foaming agent and a foaming aid before foaming, and heated under pressure. A small amount of odorous ammonia gas in the gas generated by the foaming agent in the chemical reaction of gasification is sealed in the EVA bubble. It takes a while to diverge. Therefore, the newly purchased foamed EVA Taekwondo mats will be opened for a few days, and there is no big problem. Ammonia is not poisoned at all, and many of the foaming agents in our usual foods will be produced. New shoes like the ones you buy will have a taste, because the soles are also made of EVA plastic foam, and the taste will be gone. A simple and effective method is to add an appropriate amount of EVA deodorant to the production of EVA Taekwondo mats. Through specific chemical enthalpy and action, it can effectively clear the various odors of EVA in processing and use, and is safe and environmentally friendly. Of course, the cost will also increase!

EVA resin is environmentally friendly. The smell may not be formal, or the reason for packaging. EVA is an ethylene-vinyl acetate (vinyl acetate) copolymer which is obtained by copolymerization of ethylene (E) and vinyl acetate (VA), and is English name: Ethylene Vinyl Acetate, abbreviated as EVA, or E/VAC. Generally, the content of vinyl acetate (VA) is 5% to 40%. Compared with polyethylene, EVA has reduced vinylation due to the introduction of vinyl acetate monomer in the molecular chain, improving flexibility, impact resistance, filler compatibility and heat sealing performance. In general, the performance of EVA resins depends primarily on the amount of vinyl acetate on the molecular chain. Due to the adjustable composition ratio to meet different application requirements, the higher the content of VA content, the higher the transparency, comfort and toughness.

Experts suggest that after purchasing plastic floor mats, they should be aired in a ventilated place to make the toxic substances contained in them fully volatilized; consumers should buy such products at the supermarkets or high-quality platforms, and smell them before buying. Not necessarily non-toxic, must not buy it."
https://amzn.to/2ZXoBIC
SAFEST Non Toxic Alphabet Puzzle Mat

www.ingramcontent.com/pod-product-compliance
Lightning Source LLC
Chambersburg PA
CBHW031921270726
48655CB00007BA/3118